THE OBESITY ACT:

Decoding The Weight Loss Mysteries

By

Donald V. Schaper

DISCLAIMER

Table of Contents

CHAPTER ONE

INTRODUCTION

Obesity is a medical condition characterized by an excessive accumulation of body fat that can negatively impact an individual's health. It is typically defined as having a body mass index (BMI) of 30 or higher, although this can vary depending on factors such as muscle mass and body composition.

The introduction to obesity typically outlines the prevalence and impact of this condition on individuals and society. According to the World Health Organization (WHO), obesity has nearly tripled worldwide since 1975. In 2016, more than 1.nine billion adults had been overweight, and over 650 million had been obese. In the United States, approximately 40% of adults are considered obese.Obesity is related to a huge variety of terrible fitness outcomes, consisting of an extended risk of type 2 diabetes, cardiovascular disease, stroke, certain types of cancer, and other chronic conditions. It can also negatively impact mental health and quality of life.

This book will discuss the potential causes and risk factors associated with this condition. These include genetic factors, environmental factors such as diet and physical activity, hormonal imbalances, and certain medical conditions or medications.

The introduction also outlines the various strategies for managing and treating obesity, including lifestyle changes such as diet and exercise, medication, and in severe cases, bariatric surgery.

The introduction to obesity provides an overview of this complex and multifaceted condition, highlighting its impact on individuals and society and outlining the various approaches for addressing it.

The introduction to obesity serves as a starting point for understanding the nature and impact of this condition. It sets the stage for the rest of the discussion by providing a broad overview of the topic.

One of the key aspects of the introduction is highlighting the prevalence of obesity and its negative health consequences. The statistics on the rise of obesity around the world are startling and underscore the need for greater attention and action to address the issue. By outlining the many health risks associated with obesity, the introduction can help to raise awareness of the importance of preventing and treating this condition.

In addition to discussing the prevalence and impact of obesity, the introduction may also delve into the potential causes and risk factors associated with the condition. This can help readers to better understand the many factors that contribute to obesity, from genetics to lifestyle and environmental factors.

The introduction can help to set expectations for the rest of the discussion by providing an overview of the various strategies for managing and treating obesity. By highlighting the range of options available, readers can gain a better understanding of the complexity of the issue and the many approaches that may be needed to address it.

The Obesity Epidemic

The obesity epidemic is a term used to describe the widespread increase in the number of people who are overweight or obese. The World Health Organization (WHO) defines obesity as having a body mass index (BMI) of 30 or higher, while being overweight is defined as a BMI of 25 or higher.

The obesity epidemic is a global phenomenon affecting both developed and developing countries. In recent decades, the prevalence of obesity has increased dramatically. According to WHO, in 2016 more than 1.nine billion adults were overweight, and over 650 million have been obese. In the United States, nearly 40% of adults are considered obese, and the rates of childhood obesity have also risen significantly.

CHAPTER TWO

UNDERSTANDING THE CAUSES OF OBESITY

Understanding the causes of obesity is an important step towards addressing this complex and widespread issue. There are many factors that contribute to the development of obesity, including genetic, environmental, and behavioral factors.

One of the primary causes of obesity is an imbalance between energy intake and energy expenditure. When an individual consumes more calories than their body requires for energy, the excess calories are stored as fat, leading to weight gain over time. This can occur due to a variety of factors, including a diet that is high in calories, low in nutrients, and lacking in fiber, as well as a sedentary lifestyle that involves little physical activity.

1. Genetic factors play a role in an individual's susceptibility to obesity. Some people may have a genetic predisposition to gaining weight more easily than others due to differences in metabolism, appetite, and energy expenditure.

Genetics can also play a role in the development of obesity. Studies have shown that genes can influence an individual's metabolism, appetite, and energy expenditure, making some people more susceptible to weight gain than others. However, genetics alone do not determine whether an individual will develop obesity. Environmental and lifestyle factors also play a significant role.

2. Environmental factors also play a significant role in the development of obesity. For example, access to healthy foods and safe places to exercise can influence an individual's ability to maintain a healthy weight. Individuals living in low-income neighborhoods may have limited access to healthy foods, making it more difficult to make healthy food choices. In addition, environmental factors such as stress, lack of sleep, and exposure to certain chemicals may also contribute to weight gain and obesity.

Environmental factors such as access to healthy foods and safe places to exercise can also influence an individual's risk for obesity. For example, individuals living in low-income neighborhoods may have limited access to healthy foods, which can lead to reliance on fast food and other unhealthy options. In addition, a lack of safe and accessible places to exercise may discourage physical activity, making it more difficult to maintain a healthy weight.

3. Behavioral factors also contribute to the development of obesity. For example, eating habits and physical activity levels can have a significant impact on weight. Overeating, frequent snacking, and consumption of high-calorie, low-nutrient foods can contribute to weight gain. Similarly, a lack of physical activity can contribute to weight gain by reducing energy expenditure and promoting the accumulation of body fat.

Behavioral factors, such as eating habits and physical activity levels, can also contribute to the development of obesity. Overeating, frequent snacking, and consumption of high-calorie, low-nutrient foods can all contribute to weight gain. Similarly, a lack of physical activity can lead to a decrease in energy expenditure, making it more difficult to maintain a healthy weight.

In order to address the complex causes of obesity, it is important to develop a multifaceted approach that addresses both individual and environmental factors. This may include interventions such as promoting healthy eating habits and regular physical activity, improving access to healthy foods and safe places to exercise, and implementing policies that support healthy behaviors. By addressing the many factors that contribute to obesity, it is possible to help individuals and communities to achieve and maintain a healthy weight.

CHAPTER THREE

THE ROLE OF INSULIN IN WEIGHT GAIN

Insulin is a hormone that is responsible for regulating the amount of glucose (sugar) in the bloodstream. When an individual consumes carbohydrates, insulin is released by the pancreas to help transport glucose into cells where it can be used for energy. Insulin also plays a critical role in the storage and breakdown of fat in the body.

When insulin levels are high, the body is in an anabolic state, meaning it is focused on storing energy rather than burning it. This can lead to an increase in fat storage and weight gain. Consuming a diet that is high in refined carbohydrates, such as white bread, pasta, and sugary snacks, can cause insulin levels to spike, leading to an increase in fat storage.

In addition to dietary factors, insulin resistance can also contribute to weight gain. Insulin resistance occurs when the body's cells become less responsive to insulin, making it more difficult for glucose to be transported into cells. This can lead to high blood sugar levels, increased insulin production, and an increased risk of weight gain and obesity.

Consuming a diet that is high in refined carbohydrates, such as white bread, pasta, and sugary snacks, can cause insulin levels to spike, leading to an increase in fat storage. Similarly, consuming large quantities of sugary drinks can also lead to spikes in insulin levels and increased fat storage.

Insulin resistance is often associated with a sedentary lifestyle and a diet high in refined carbohydrates and saturated fats. Other factors that can contribute to insulin resistance include obesity, aging, and genetics.

To prevent weight gain associated with insulin resistance, it is important to consume a balanced diet that is low in refined carbohydrates and high in fiber-rich foods, such as fruits, vegetables, and whole grains. Regular exercise can also help to improve insulin sensitivity and reduce the risk of weight gain. In some cases, medication or other medical interventions may be necessary to manage insulin resistance and prevent weight gain.

Overall, maintaining healthy insulin levels is important for maintaining a healthy weight and reducing the risk of obesity-related health conditions. By consuming a balanced diet, engaging in regular exercise, and managing insulin resistance, it is possible to support healthy insulin levels and prevent weight gain.

CHAPTER FOUR

THE SCIENCE OF FAT STORAGE AND RELEASE

The science of fat storage and release involves complex metabolic processes in the body that are controlled by various hormones and enzymes. Understanding how these processes work can provide insight into how the body regulates weight and can inform strategies for weight loss and management.

When an individual consumes food, the body breaks down the carbohydrates, fats, and proteins into their component parts. Carbohydrates are broken down into glucose, which is used as a primary source of energy by the body. Excess glucose that is not immediately used by the body is stored in the liver and muscles as glycogen.

Fats, on the other hand, are broken down into fatty acids and glycerol. These components can be used by the body for energy production or stored in adipose tissue (fat cells) for later use. The process of storing fat is called lipogenesis, and it is controlled by a hormone called insulin.

Insulin is released by the pancreas in response to high levels of glucose in the bloodstream. When insulin levels are high, the body is in an anabolic state, meaning it is focused on storing energy rather than burning it. Insulin promotes the uptake of glucose and fatty acids into cells for storage as glycogen and fat, respectively.

When the body needs energy, it can release stored fat from adipose tissue in a process called lipolysis. This process is controlled by a hormone called glucagon, which is released by the pancreas when blood sugar levels are low. Glucagon signals the body to break down stored glycogen and fat to provide energy for the body.

The release of fat from adipose tissue is also regulated by other hormones, such as leptin and adiponectin. Leptin is a hormone produced by adipose tissue that helps to regulate hunger and metabolism. When levels of leptin are high, it signals the brain that the body has enough energy and suppresses hunger. Adiponectin, on the other hand, helps to regulate insulin sensitivity and fat metabolism.

Factors that can contribute to increased fat storage and decreased fat release include a sedentary lifestyle, a diet high in refined carbohydrates and saturated fats, and insulin resistance. Insulin resistance occurs when the body's cells become less responsive to insulin, making it more difficult for glucose and fatty acids to be transported into cells. This can lead to high blood sugar levels, increased insulin production, and an increased risk of weight gain and obesity.

To support healthy fat storage and release, it is important to maintain a balanced diet that is low in refined carbohydrates and high in fiber-rich foods, such as fruits, vegetables, and whole grains. Regular exercise can also help to improve insulin sensitivity and promote the release of stored fat for energy. In some cases, medication or other medical interventions may be necessary to manage insulin resistance and support healthy weight management.

The science of fat storage and release is complex and involves multiple hormones and metabolic processes in the body. Understanding these processes can help inform strategies for healthy weight management and support overall health and wellbeing.

CHAPTER FIVE

THE IMPORTANCE OF MEAL TIMING AND FREQUENCY

The importance of meal timing and frequency refers to the practice of when and how often one consumes meals throughout the day. This has been shown to have significant effects on metabolism, weight management, and overall health.

One key aspect of meal timing is circadian rhythm. The body has a natural internal clock that regulates various physiological processes, including metabolism. Eating meals at regular intervals and at consistent times of day can help to regulate the body's circadian rhythm, leading to more efficient energy metabolism and improved health outcomes.

Research has also shown that the frequency of meals can impact metabolism and weight management. Some studies suggest that consuming multiple small meals throughout the day, rather than a few large meals, can help to regulate blood sugar levels, improve insulin sensitivity, and support healthy weight management.

Additionally, the timing of meals can affect hormone levels, particularly insulin and leptin. Insulin is released in response to carbohydrate consumption and signals the body to store glucose and fat. Leptin is a hormone that regulates hunger and satiety, and its levels fluctuate in response to meals. Eating meals that are high in carbohydrates, particularly in the evening, can lead to increased insulin levels and decreased leptin levels, which can contribute to weight gain and other health issues.

Furthermore, research has shown that skipping meals, particularly breakfast, can have negative effects on metabolism and weight management. Skipping meals can lead to decreased metabolic rate and increased insulin resistance, which can make it more difficult to lose weight and maintain a healthy weight.

In addition to the timing and frequency of meals, the content of meals is also important. Consuming a balanced diet that is rich in whole foods, including fruits, vegetables, whole grains, and lean proteins, can help to support healthy weight management and overall health.

Overall, the importance of meal timing and frequency cannot be overstated. Consistent meal timing, consuming meals at regular intervals, and consuming a balanced diet can help to regulate metabolism, support healthy weight management, and promote overall health and wellbeing.

CHAPTER SIX

THE BENEFITS OF INTERMITTENT FASTING

Intermittent fasting is a dietary approach that involves alternating periods of fasting with periods of normal eating. There are several different types of intermittent fasting, but the most common method involves restricting food intake for a set period of time each day, such as 16 hours of fasting followed by 8 hours of eating.

There are many potential benefits of intermittent fasting, including:

Weight loss: Intermittent fasting has been shown to be an effective weight loss strategy. By restricting food intake, the body is forced to use stored fat for energy, leading to decreased body fat and weight loss.

Improved insulin sensitivity: Intermittent fasting can improve insulin sensitivity, which is important for maintaining healthy blood sugar levels and preventing type 2 diabetes.

Reduced inflammation: Intermittent fasting has been shown to reduce inflammation in the body, which can help to prevent chronic diseases such as heart disease, cancer, and Alzheimer's.

Improved brain function: Intermittent fasting has been shown to improve cognitive function and protect against age-related cognitive decline.

Longevity: Intermittent fasting has been shown to increase lifespan in animal studies, and there is some evidence to suggest that it may have similar effects in humans.

Convenience: Intermittent fasting can be a convenient way to manage food intake, as it eliminates the need to constantly plan and prepare meals throughout the day.

Improved eating habits: Intermittent fasting can help to promote healthier eating habits by encouraging individuals to consume more nutrient-dense foods during their eating periods.

It's important to note that intermittent fasting may not be appropriate for everyone, particularly those with certain health conditions or who are pregnant or breastfeeding. Additionally, it's important to maintain a balanced and nutritious diet during eating periods to ensure that the body is getting the nutrients it needs.

Intermittent fasting can be a safe and effective way to promote weight loss, improve health, and enhance overall wellbeing. However, it's important to speak with a healthcare professional before starting an intermittent fasting regimen to ensure that it is safe and appropriate for your individual needs.

CHAPTER SEVEN

THE MYTH OF CALORIES IN, CALORIES OUT

The "calories in, calories out" model of weight loss is based on the idea that weight gain occurs when an individual consumes more calories than they burn, and weight loss occurs when they burn more calories than they consume. This model is often oversimplified, and does not take into account a variety of other factors that can impact weight gain and loss.

The "calories in, calories out" model of weight loss assumes that a calorie is a calorie, regardless of its source. However, research has shown that different macronutrients (protein, carbohydrates, and fat) can have different effects on the body. For example, a calorie from protein can increase satiety and boost metabolism, while a calorie from refined carbohydrates can cause blood sugar spikes and crashes, leading to increased hunger and overeating.

One of the main issues with the "calories in, calories out" model is that it assumes that all calories are equal, regardless of their source. However, research has shown that different types of calories can have different effects on the body. For example, a calorie from protein may have a different impact on metabolism than a calorie from carbohydrates or fat.

Another issue with the "calories in, calories out" model is that it does not account for individual differences in metabolism and hormone regulation. Different individuals may have different metabolic rates and respond differently to changes in calorie intake, making it difficult to predict the impact of calorie restriction on weight loss.

Additionally, the "calories in, calories out" model does not consider the impact of factors such as stress, sleep, and gut health on weight gain and loss. These factors can all have a significant impact on metabolism and hormone regulation, and can therefore impact weight loss efforts.

The efficiency of the "calories in, calories out" weight loss approach can also be impacted by individual variances in metabolism and hormone regulation. For example, persons with slower metabolisms may require fewer calories to maintain their weight, making it more difficult for them to establish a calorie deficit by diet alone. Similarly, hormonal imbalances, such as insulin resistance or thyroid dysfunction, can alter metabolism and make it harder to lose weight.

Furthermore, it is impossible to disregard the influence of elements like stress, sleep, and gut health on weight growth and reduction. Persistent stress can lead to high levels of the hormone cortisol, which can stimulate hunger and lead to weight gain. Hormone regulation problems, increased hunger, and cravings have all been connected to poor sleep quality. Moreover, an unbalanced gut bacterial population can cause inflammation and insulin resistance, both of which might hinder your attempts to lose weight.

The "calories in, calories out" model does not take into account the importance of food quality and nutrient density for weight loss. While a calorie deficit is necessary for weight loss, consuming a diet rich in whole, nutrient-dense foods can support weight loss efforts by promoting satiety, reducing inflammation, and supporting metabolic function.

In summary, while the "calories in, calories out" model can be a useful tool for weight loss, it should not be viewed as the only factor to consider. Other factors such as food quality, nutrient density, individual differences in metabolism and hormone regulation, and lifestyle factors like stress and sleep should also be taken into account when attempting to lose weight.

CHAPTER EIGHT

HOW TO BREAK THE
CYCLE OF OBESITY

Breaking the cycle of obesity can be a challenging
and complex process, but there are several key steps
that can be taken to achieve long-term weight loss
and improve overall health. Here are some
strategies that can be helpful:

Adopt a whole foods, nutrient-dense diet: Focus
on eating whole foods that are rich in nutrients and
avoid processed foods that are high in sugar, salt,
and unhealthy fats. Eating a balanced diet that

includes plenty of vegetables, fruits, whole grains, lean proteins, and healthy fats can help to improve overall health and support weight loss.

Address underlying health conditions: Certain health conditions, such as insulin resistance or hypothyroidism, can make it more difficult to lose weight. It's important to work with a healthcare provider to identify and address any underlying health issues that may be contributing to weight gain.

Practice mindful eating: Mindful eating involves paying attention to hunger and fullness cues and eating slowly and without distraction. This can help to prevent overeating and improve overall food choices

.

Increase physical activity: Regular physical activity is important for weight loss and overall health. Aim for at least 30 minutes of moderate-intensity exercise most days of the week, and incorporate both aerobic exercise and strength training into your routine.

Get enough sleep: Sleep is important for regulating hormones that control appetite and metabolism, so getting enough sleep is essential for weight loss. Aim for 7-9 hours of sleep per night, and establish a regular sleep routine to improve sleep quality.Manage strain: Chronic strain can make contributions to weight benefit and make it tough to lose weight. Finding healthy ways to manage stress, such as practicing mindfulness, yoga, or meditation, can be helpful for weight loss and overall health.

Seek support: Losing weight can be challenging, and having support from friends, family, or a healthcare provider can be helpful. Consider joining a weight loss support group, working with a registered dietitian, or seeking guidance from a healthcare provider to help you achieve your weight loss goals.

By adopting these strategies, it is possible to break the cycle of obesity and achieve long-term weight loss and improved health. However, it is important to remember that weight loss is a journey, and it may take time and effort to achieve your goals.

CHAPTER NINE

STRATEGIES FOR SUSTAINABLE WEIGHT LOSS

Sustainable weight reduction entails making lifestyle modifications that may be maintained over the lengthy term. Here are some strategies for sustainable weight loss:

Set realistic goals: Setting realistic goals can help to prevent feelings of frustration and failure. Aim to lose 1-2 pounds per week, and focus on making small changes that can be maintained over time.

Eat a balanced, nutrient-dense diet: A balanced diet that is rich in nutrients can help to support weight loss and improve overall health. Focus on eating plenty of vegetables, fruits, whole grains, lean proteins, and healthy fats, and avoid processed and sugary foods.

Practice portion control: Paying attention to portion sizes can help to prevent overeating and promote weight loss. Use smaller plates, measure out servings, and eat slowly to give your body time to register fullness.

Keep a food diary: Keeping a food diary can help to increase awareness of eating habits and provide accountability. Write down what you eat and drink, as well as how you feel before and after meals.

Stay hydrated: Drinking plenty of water can help to prevent overeating and improve overall health. Aim for at least 8 cups of water per day, and limit sugary drinks.

Be physically active: Regular physical activity is important for weight loss and overall health. Aim for at least 30 minutes of moderate-intensity exercise most days of the week, and incorporate both aerobic exercise and strength training into your routine.

Get enough sleep: Sleep is important for regulating hormones that control appetite and metabolism, so getting enough sleep is essential for weight loss. Aim for 7-nine hours of sleep in line with night, and set up an ordinary sleep routine to enhance sleep quality.

Practice stress management: Chronic stress can contribute to weight gain and make it difficult to lose weight. Finding healthy ways to manage stress, such as practicing mindfulness, yoga, or meditation, can be helpful for weight loss and overall health.

Seek support: Losing weight can be challenging, and having support from friends, family, or a healthcare provider can be helpful. Consider joining a weight loss support group, working with a registered dietitian, or seeking guidance from a healthcare provider to help you achieve your weight loss goals.

By adopting these strategies, it is certain to achieve sustainable weight loss and improve overall health. However, it's important to remember that weight loss is a journey and that small changes over time can lead to long-term success.

CONCLUSION

A thorough guide to comprehending the factors contributing to obesity and effective weight loss techniques is The Obesity Act: Understanding the Weight Loss Secrets. The book offers a more complex understanding of the intricate hormonal and metabolic processes that control fat storage and release, challenging the conventional belief that weight gain is simply a matter of consuming more calories than you expend. Treating insulin resistance through changes in food and lifestyle is critical for attaining sustainable weight loss. People can end the cycle of obesity and get to a healthier weight by implementing tactics like intermittent fasting, meal planning, frequency, and exercise.